RAISING VEGAN BABIES

Essential Tips, Nutrition Strategies, and Recipes for Parenting Healthy and Happy Kids on a Plant-Based Diet from Infancy to Toddlerhood

By

Sharon G. Brown

TABLE OF CONTENT

INTRODUCTION

Welcome to the wonderful journey of vegan parenting! Whether you are a novice parent, anticipating parenthood, or contemplating adopting a plant-based lifestyle for your child, this book is designed to provide comprehensive guidance and assistance throughout the entire process. Choosing to raise your child on a vegan diet demonstrates your dedication to promoting well-being, empathy, and environmental responsibility. It is a way that not only promotes the physical and emotional health of your child but also contributes to a more compassionate and environmentally sustainable world.

The advantages of adopting a vegan diet have become widely acknowledged in recent years, supported by substantial research and approved by healthcare experts. Plant-based diets, abundant in fruits, vegetables, whole grains, nuts, and legumes, supply all the vital nutrients required for development and growth. In addition, they are linked to a reduced likelihood of developing chronic illnesses, making them a healthful option for people of all age groups.

Parenting a vegan infant has unique challenges and opportunities. As a parent, you aim to guarantee that your child has all the essential nutrients for ideal growth and development. The purpose of this book is to clarify the principles of vegan nutrition and equip you with the information and resources necessary to effectively supply your child with proper nourishment from infancy to toddlerhood and beyond.

In "Raising Vegan Babies" you will find:

Nutritional Guidance: Comprehensive insights into vital nutrients, strategies for fulfilling your child's dietary requirements, and recommendations for achieving well-rounded and diverse meals.

Practical Guidance: Techniques for initiating the consumption of solid foods, addressing common issues such as selective eating, and managing social circumstances as a family following a vegan lifestyle.

Recipes and Meal Plans: These recipes and plans are tailored to meet your kids nutritional requirements, guaranteeing both tasty and nourishing meals.

This book aims to serve as a valuable resource and a source of inspiration as you begin your journey into vegan parenting.

With the knowledge you gain from this book, you will be able to confidently make decisions that are best for your baby. Whether you're a first-time parent or planning to go vegan with your family, this book will help you raise a compassionate and healthy baby.

CHAPTER ONE

Why Select a Plant-Based Diet for Your Child?

Choosing a plant-based diet for your child can have significant and long-term benefits for their health, well-being, and the environment. Here are some compelling reasons why a vegan diet may be an ideal choice for parenting your child:

1. Optimized Nutrition

A well-planned vegan diet can give your child all of the nutrients he or she requires for healthy development. Plant-based foods contain high levels of vitamins, minerals, antioxidants, and fiber, all of which are essential for overall health. Plant foods contain key nutrients such as protein, iron, calcium, and omega-3 fatty acids, ensuring your child's nutrition is balanced and thorough.

2. Disease Prevention.

According to studies, a plant-based diet can lower the risk of chronic diseases like heart disease, diabetes, and certain malignancies. By emphasizing whole, nutrient-dense meals, you may help your kid develop good eating habits that support long-term wellness and lower the chance of developing lifestyle-related diseases later in life.

3. Healthy Weight Management.

Children raised on a plant-based diet are less likely to become obese. Plant meals are often lower in calories and richer in fiber, which helps to regulate appetite and promotes good weight management. This can pave the way for a lifetime of healthy eating and weight management.

4. Environmental Impact.

A vegan diet is one of the most efficient methods to lessen your environmental impact. Animal agriculture significantly contributes to greenhouse gas emissions, deforestation, and water consumption. Raising your child on a plant-based diet benefits the environment and helps to preserve it for future generations.

5. Ethical considerations

A vegan diet promotes compassion and respect for animals. Teaching your child the value of kindness to animals helps promote empathy and a sense of responsibility for all living things. This ethical basis can mold their personality and impact their decisions throughout their lives.

6. Culinary Diversity.

A plant-based diet promotes the exploration of a diverse range of foods and cuisines. Incorporating different fruits, vegetables, grains, legumes, nuts, and seeds into your child's diet exposes them to a variety of flavors and sensations. This can help children improve their palate and become more willing to try new meals.

7. Support for Immunity

Plants are high in antioxidants and phytochemicals, which boost the immune system. A fruit and vegetable-rich diet will help your child fight illnesses and stay healthy.

8. Promoting Lifelong Healthy Habits.

Raising your child on a vegan diet instills healthy eating habits from an early age. Prioritizing complete, plant-based foods sets a good example and promotes long-term mindful eating habits.

Choosing a plant-based diet for your child is an effective method to improve their health, develop ethical values, and save the environment. With careful preparation and a focus on nutrient-dense foods, you can ensure that your child has all they need to flourish. Embrace the vegan parenting path with confidence, knowing you are positively impacting your child's future and the world they live in.

Essential Nutrients for Growing Infants and Toddlers

Ensuring that your infant or toddler receives all of the necessary nutrients is critical for their growth and development. A well-planned vegan diet can provide these nutrients; however, it is critical to understand which nutrients are required and how to incorporate them into your child's diet. Here are the essential nutrients and their plant-based sources:

1. Protein.

Protein is essential for growth, muscle development, and general health. It can be present in many plant-based meals.

Sources include lentils, chickpeas, beans, tofu, tempeh, quinoa, nuts, seeds, and nut butters.

2. Iron

Iron is required for proper blood and brain development. Plant-based iron (non-heme iron) is most readily absorbed when combined with vitamin C-rich meals, bell peppers, oranges, strawberries, and broccoli.

Sources include lentils, chickpeas, beans, quinoa, tofu, spinach, fortified cereals, pumpkin seeds, and blackstrap molasses.

3. Calcium

Calcium is essential for healthy bones and teeth. Although dairy is a prominent source, there are other plant-based alternatives.

Sources include fortified plant milks (almond, soy, and oat), orange juice, tofu, broccoli, kale, bok choy, almonds, and tahini.

4. Vitamin D

Vitamin D promotes bone health and immunological function. It might be difficult to get enough from food alone, especially in areas with little sunlight.

Fortified plant milks, fortified orange juice, and vitamins (see a pediatrician for recommended dosage).

5. Vitamin B-12

Vitamin B12 is required for nerve function and the formation of red blood cells. It does not occur naturally in plant foods, thus supplementation is required.

Sources include enriched plant milks, cereals, nutritional yeast, and supplements.

6. Omega 3 Fatty Acids

Omega-3 fatty acids are essential to brain growth and function. While fish is a popular source, there are plant-based alternatives as well.

Sources include flaxseeds, chia seeds, hemp seeds, walnuts, and algae-based supplements.

7. Zinc

Zinc helps the immune system and promotes cellular growth.

Sources include legumes, chickpeas, lentils, beans, tofu, nuts, seeds, and whole grains.

8. Iodine.

Iodine is necessary for thyroid function and brain development.

Sources: Iodized salt and seaweed (in moderation to prevent overconsumption).

9. Fiber

Fiber promotes intestinal health and prevents constipation.

Sources include fruits, vegetables, whole grains, legumes, nuts, and seeds.

10. Vitamin A.

Vitamin A promotes vision, immunological function, and skin health.

Sources include carrots, sweet potatoes, butternut squash, dark leafy greens, and apricots.

CHAPTER TWO

Balancing a Vegan Diet for Babies and Toddlers

To ensure a balanced vegan diet for your developing child, consider the following suggestions:

Variety: Offer a wide range of foods to fulfill all nutrient needs. Different foods have different nutrients; thus, variety is essential.

Fortified foods: Fortified foods can help you achieve your nutritional needs, notably vitamins B12, D, and iron.

Regular Meal and Snacks: Provide your child with regular meals and snacks to ensure they get adequate calories and nutrients throughout the day.

Monitor growth: To ensure that your child's growth and development are on track, check in with your pediatrician on a regular basis.

A well-planned vegan diet can cover all of the nutritional requirements of developing infants and toddlers. Understanding the key elements and incorporating a range of plant-based foods will guarantee that your child receives the nourishment they require for healthy growth and development. Always visit a pediatrician or qualified nutritionist to create a diet plan that is tailored to your child's individual needs.

Macronutrients: Proteins, Carbs, and Fats

Macronutrients are the nutrients that your body requires in significant quantities to provide energy and sustain basic activities. Proteins, carbs, and fats are the three most common macronutrients. Each has a particular impact on your child's growth and development.

Proteins:

- Essential for tissue growth and repair.

- Enzymes, hormones, and other bodily components require it to function properly.

➢ Muscles, skin, and organs rely on amino acids for their construction.

Plant-Based Sources:

- Legumes which include lentils, chickpeas, black beans, and kidney beans.

- Soy products which include tofu, tempeh, and edamame.

- Whole grains which include quinoa, amaranth, and bulgur.

- Nuts and seeds which include almonds, chia seeds, hemp seeds, and pumpkin seeds.

- Nut butters which include peanut butter, almond butter, and sunflower seed butter.

Tips:

Combine various plant-based protein sources to achieve a full amino acid profile.

Include protein-rich meals in every meal to meet your daily protein needs.

Carbohydrates:

- The main source of energy for the body.

- Important for brain function, particularly in developing infants.

- Provides fiber, which assists digestion and prevents constipation.

Plant-Based Sources:

> Whole grains which include brown rice, oatmeal, barley, whole wheat pasta, and whole grain bread.

> Vegetables which include sweet potatoes, potatoes, carrots, and corn.

> Fruits which include bananas, apples, berries, and mangoes.

> Legumes which include beans, lentils, and peas.

Other sources include quinoa, bulgur, and millet.

Tips:

- To get the most nutrients, eat whole, unprocessed carbs.

- Include a variety of colored fruits and vegetables to guarantee a balanced intake of vitamins and minerals.

Fat:

- Delivers a focused source of energy.

- Essential for brain growth and function.

- Facilitates the absorption of fat-soluble vitamins (A, D, E, and K).

Plant-Based Sources:

➤ Nuts and seeds include walnuts, flaxseed, chia seeds, and hemp seeds.

➤ Healthy oils include olive oil, coconut oil, and avocado oil.

➢ Avocado: High in monounsaturated fats.

➢ Coconut products include coconut milk and coconut cream.

➢ Nut Butters: Peanut butter and almond butter.

Tips:

- Include a source of healthy fat in each meal to promote overall wellness.

- To keep your calorie consumption in check, pay attention to portion sizes.

Functions of Vitamins, Minerals and Their Sources

Micronutrients are vitamins and minerals that the body needs in little amounts yet are essential for many biological activities, growth, and disease prevention.

Vitamins A:

Role: Critical to vision, immunological function, and skin health.

Carrots, sweet potatoes, apricots, and dark leafy greens are all good sources.

Vitamin B 12:

Role: Essential for nerve function and red blood cell formation.

Sources include fortified plant milks, nutritional yeast, and supplements.

Vitamin C:

Supports the immune system, improves iron absorption, and promotes skin health.

Citrus fruits, bell peppers, strawberries, and broccoli are some of the sources.

Vitamin D:

Role: Critical to bone health and immunological function.

Sources include fortified plant milks, orange juice, supplements, and sun exposure.

Vitamin E:

Functions as an antioxidant, protecting cells from harm.

Sources: Nuts, seeds, spinach, broccoli, and sunflower oil.

Vitamin K:

Role: Required for blood clotting and bone health.

Sources include kale, spinach, broccoli, and Brussels sprouts.

Minerals

Calcium:

Role: Essential for bone and tooth health.

Sources include fortified plant milks, tofu, broccoli, kale, and almonds.

Iron:

Role: Required for the formation of hemoglobin and overall oxygen transport in the body.

Sources include lentils, chickpeas, beans, quinoa, spinach, and fortified cereals.

Magnesium:

Role: Promotes muscle and nerve function, as well as energy production.

Sources include nuts, seeds, whole grains, legumes, and leafy green vegetables.

Zinc:

Role: Promotes immunological function and cellular proliferation.

Sources include legumes, chickpeas, lentils, beans, nuts, seeds, and whole grains.

Iodine:

Role: Required for thyroid function and brain development.

Sources: iodized salt and seaweed (in moderation).

Omega 3 Fatty Acids:

Role: Critical to brain growth and function.

Sources include flaxseeds, chia seeds, hemp seeds, walnuts, and algae-based supplements.

Understanding the roles and sources of macronutrients and key micronutrients is critical when designing a healthy vegan diet for your developing child. By incorporating a range of nutrient-dense plant-based meals, you may ensure that your child gets all of the nutrients he or she needs for healthy growth and development. Always work with a doctor or trained dietitian to create a diet plan that is tailored to your child's needs and ensures they are fulfilling their nutritional requirements.

CHAPTER THREE

Vegan Nutrition While Pregnant

Pregnancy necessitates higher nutritional requirements to maintain the health and development of both the mother and the baby. A carefully planned vegan diet can provide all of the nutrients required for a healthy pregnancy. Here are the important concerns and nutritional sources:

Essential Nutrients:

- ➤ **Protein**

Role: Promotes fetal growth and maternal tissue development.

Sources include lentils, chickpeas, beans, tofu, tempeh, quinoa, nuts, seeds, and nut butters.

➢ **Iron**

Role: Required for increased blood volume and oxygen transportation. Vitamin C-rich foods, such as bell peppers, oranges, and strawberries, improve iron absorption.

Sources include lentils, chickpeas, beans, tofu, spinach, quinoa, fortified cereals, and pumpkin seeds.

➢ **Calcium**

Role: Critical to prenatal bone growth and mother bone health.

Sources include fortified plant milks (almond, soy, and oat), fortified orange juice, tofu, broccoli, kale, bok choy, almonds, and tahini.

> **Vitamin D**

Role: Promotes bone health and immunological function.

Sources include fortified plant milks, fortified orange juice, and supplements (see your doctor for the proper amount).

Vitamin B 12

Role: Required for nerve activity and red blood cell formation.

Sources include fortified plant milks, nutritional yeast, and supplements.

➢ **Folate (vitamin B9)**

Role: Essential for DNA synthesis and avoiding neural tube abnormalities.

Sources include leafy green vegetables, legumes, fortified cereals, oranges, avocados, and supplements.

➢ **Omega 3 Fatty Acids**

Role: Critical for the brain and ocular development of the fetus.

Sources include flaxseeds, chia seeds, hemp seeds, walnuts, and algae-based supplements.

➢ **Zinc**

Role: Promotes immunological function and cellular proliferation.

Sources include legumes, chickpeas, lentils, beans, nuts, seeds, and whole grains.

> **Iodine**

Role: Required for thyroid function and brain development.

Sources include iodized salt and seaweed (in moderation).

> **Fiber**

Role: Promotes digestion and prevents constipation, which is frequent during pregnancy.

Sources include fruits, vegetables, whole grains, legumes, nuts, and seeds.

Practical Tips for Expecting Mothers

- Balanced Meals: Make sure each meal has a combination of protein, healthy fats, and complex carbohydrates.

- Eat modest, regular meals and snacks to keep your energy levels stable and combat nausea.

- Hydration: Drink plenty of water to stay hydrated and promote increased blood volume.

- Supplements: Take a prenatal vitamin to fill any nutritional shortages, particularly vitamin B12, vitamin D, and DHA (a kind of omega-3 fatty acid). Before beginning any new supplement regimen, always consult with your doctor.

Breastfeeding with a Plant-Based Diet

Breastfeeding gives vital nutrients to the baby and strengthens their immune system. When properly planned, a vegan diet can meet the nutritional needs of both the mother and the breastfeeding baby.

Essential Nutrients:

> **Protein**

Supports milk production, as well as maternal tissue growth and healing.

Sources include lentils, chickpeas, beans, tofu, tempeh, quinoa, nuts, seeds, and nut butters.

> **Calcium**

Role: Crucial to the baby's bone development and the mother's bone health.

Sources include fortified plant milks, orange juice, tofu, broccoli, kale, bok choy, almonds, and tahini.

> **Vitamin B 12**

Role: Critical to the baby's neurological development and the mother's energy levels.

Sources include fortified plant milks, nutritional yeast, and supplements.

> **Vitamin D**

Role: Promotes bone health in both mother and infant.

Sources include fortified plant milks, fortified orange juice, and supplements (see your doctor for the proper amount).

> **Iron**

Role: Prevents anemia in the mother and promotes baby growth.

Sources include lentils, chickpeas, beans, tofu, spinach, quinoa, fortified cereals, and pumpkin seeds.

> **Omega 3 Fatty Acids**

Role: Critical to the baby's brain and vision development.

Sources include flaxseeds, chia seeds, hemp seeds, walnuts, and algae-based supplements.

➢ **Zinc**

Role: aids in immunological function and tissue repair.

Sources include legumes, chickpeas, lentils, beans, nuts, seeds, and whole grains.

➢ **Iodine**

Role: Critical for thyroid function and newborn brain development.

Sources: iodized salt and seaweed (in moderation).

➢ **Hydration**

Role: Essential for milk production and maternal health.

Sources include water, herbal teas, soups, and hydrating fruits and vegetables.

Practical Tips

- Nutrient-Dense Foods: To achieve your nutritional demands, eat entire, nutrient-dense foods.

- Eat regular meals and snacks to stay energized and promote milk production.

- Hydration: Drink plenty of drinks to stay hydrated and promote milk production.

- Consider taking a prenatal vitamin or a breastfeeding-specific supplement, including vitamin B12, vitamin D, and DHA. Before using any new supplements, consult with your doctor.

Monitor your baby's growth and development, and schedule regular check-ups with your pediatrician to ensure they are thriving. Paying attention to these critical nutrients and following these practical tips can help you and your baby thrive on a plant-based diet during pregnancy and breastfeeding.

CHAPTER FOUR

Introduction to Plant-Based Formula

Options

Choosing the proper formula for your baby is a critical decision that will influence their health and growth. Plant-based formula alternatives are an excellent choice for parents who live a vegan lifestyle or whose newborns are allergic to cow's milk or soy.

Why Choose a Plant-Based Formula?

➢ **Health and Ethical Reasons:**

Allergies & intolerances: Some newborns are allergic to cow's milk protein or soy, thus plant-based formulas are a good option.

Vegan Lifestyle: Plant-based formulations are ethically and nutritionally appropriate for vegan families.

> **Nutritional Benefits:**

Balanced Nutrition: Plant-based formulas are intended to give complete nutrition to newborns, including all of the necessary vitamins and minerals required for growth and development.

DHA and ARA: Many plant-based formulae contain DHA (docosahexaenoic acid) and ARA (arachidonic acid), which are essential for brain and eye development.

Types of Plant-Based Formulas:

1. Soy Formula:

The most prevalent plant-based formula is made of soy protein.

Pros: Widely available, enriched with important minerals, and frequently contains DHA and ARA.

Cons: Not recommended for babies who have soy allergies or sensitivities.

2. Pea Protein-based Formula:

Made with hydrolyzed pea protein for a hypoallergenic option.

Pros: Suitable for babies allergic to cow's milk and soy, high in amino acids.

Cons: Can be more expensive and less widely available than soy-based alternatives.

3. Rice-Based Formulation:

Made with rice protein, this is another hypoallergenic choice.

Pros: Gentle on the stomach, ideal for babies with multiple food sensitivities.

Cons: Some nutrients may require further supplementation.

4. Almond-Based Formula:

Made with almond protein, this is a nut-based alternative.

Pros: High in vitamins and minerals, with a unique taste character.

Cons: Not recommended for babies with nut sensitivities, and may require additional nutrition.

Important considerations for parents:

- **Nutritional completeness**

Ensure that the formula meets newborn nutritional requirements, such as vital fatty acids, vitamins, and minerals.

- **Allergens:**

Check for probable allergies and select a formula that meets your baby's nutritional requirements and sensitivity. Always consult with your pediatrician before switching to or selecting a plant-based formula to ensure that it satisfies your baby's specific nutritional requirements.

- **Gradual Transitions:**

When switching formulas, start gradually to allow your baby's digestive system to acclimate.

- **Monitoring growth:**

Regularly consult with your pediatrician on your baby's growth and development to ensure they are thriving on the formula.

Plant-based formulas are an excellent option for babies who are allergic to cow's milk or soy, as well as families that follow a vegan diet. Plant-based formulas, with careful selection and consultation with healthcare practitioners, can provide complete and balanced nutrition to help your baby grow and develop normally.

When to Start Giving Solid Foods

According to pediatric standards, babies should start eating solid foods around 6 months. Before this, all the minerals you need come from breast milk or formula.

Signs of development:

- **Head Control:** The baby can sit up and hold their head up with only a little help.

- **Food Interest:** The baby is interested in what other people are eating.

- **Lost Tongue-Thrust Reflex:** The baby's tongue doesn't instantly push solids out of their mouth like it used to.

- **Able to Chew:** The child can put food in their back of the mouth and swallow it.

How to Start Giving Solid Foods

- Start Easy: Start with foods that only have one ingredient to check for allergies or sensitivities.

- Start with smooth purees and work your way up to mashed and then small, soft pieces as the baby gets used to eating foods.

- One Food at a Time: Every three to five days, give them a new food to see if they have any allergic responses.

- When you feed your baby, pay attention to when it tells you it's hungry or full. Do not force-feed.

- Safety: Make sure the food is the right size so no one chokes. After the first year, stay away from honey and cow's milk.

The Best Foods for Vegan Babies to Eat

First

- **Cereals with added iron:** Pick cereals made from a single grain, like rice, oats, or barley. These are great first foods because they have iron added to them.

- **Pureed veggies:** Begin with smooth veggies like peas, carrots, and sweet potatoes.

- **Fruits:** Give them fruits that have been pureed, like pears, bananas, and applesauce. The healthy fats in avocados make them even better.

- **Legumes:** Chickpeas, beans, and lentils that have been pureed are great sources of iron and protein.

- **Tofu:** You can mash soft tofu, and it has a lot of protein and iron.

- **Nut Butters:** Put almond or peanut butter thinly on a piece of bread and put it on top of cereal or purees to add protein and healthy fats.

- **Grains:** You can cook and blend quinoa and oatmeal, which are good for you grains.

Choosing Ingredients for Homemade Baby Food

For fruits, vegetables, grains, and legumes, use fresh, organic foods whenever available. Don't add salt, sugar, or spices.

Methods of Cooking: Baking or steaming keeps nutrition better than boiling. Make sure that grains and beans are cooked all the way through so that they are soft.

Pureeing: The tools you'll need to puree something are a blender, a food processor, or a hand-held immersion mixer.

Smooth purees are best for kids that are younger. For bigger babies, slowly move on to foods that are mashed or chopped very small.

Freshly made baby food can be kept in the fridge for up to 48 hours in sealed containers.

For freezing, put pieces in ice cube trays or small containers and freeze them. Put the cold food in freezer bags. Write the date and the type of food on the label. Most frozen baby food is good for three months.

Thaw cold food overnight in the fridge or in a bowl of warm water. Bring back to a lukewarm temperature. Do not put food straight in the microwave because it can make hot spots.

Hygiene: Wash your hands, dishes, and surfaces well to practice good hygiene. When you prepare and store food, always use clean tools.

Variety: Give your baby a lot of different foods to eat so that they get all the nutrients they need and to help them build their palate.

Allergen Introduction: Eating allergenic foods early (around 6 months) can help lower the chance of getting allergies, despite what other people say. Talk to your child's doctor for advice.

Watch for Reactions: If you see any of the signs of an allergic response, like rashes, swelling, or stomach problems, you should see a doctor.

CHAPTER FIVE

Creating Balanced Plant-Based Meals

Focus on plant-based protein sources, including beans, lentils, tofu, tempeh, quinoa, and edamame.

- **Iron:** Include iron-rich foods such as lentils, chickpeas, beans, tofu, spinach, and fortified cereals. Pair with vitamin C-rich foods to improve absorption.

- **Calcium:** Consume calcium-fortified plant milks (such as almond, soy, or oat milk), leafy greens (kale, bok choy), and tofu.

- **Omega-3 Fatty Acids:** Consume chia seeds, flaxseeds, hemp seeds, and walnuts.

- **Vitamin B12:** Take a B12 supplement or consume fortified foods such nutritional yeast and plant-based milk.

- **Vitamin D:** Get enough sunlight and try fortified foods or pills, especially in the winter.

- Zinc sources include legumes, seeds, nuts, and whole grains.

- **Fiber:** Eat plenty of fruits, vegetables, whole grains, legumes, nuts, and seeds.

- To structure a meal, start with a whole grain or starchy vegetable (e.g., brown rice, quinoa, sweet potatoes).

- **Protein:** Include a plant-based protein source (tofu, beans, lentils).

- **veggies:** Eat a variety of colorful veggies to obtain your vitamins, minerals, and fiber.

- **Healthy Fats:** Include avocado, nuts, and seeds.

- **Flavor:** To enhance flavor, use herbs, spices, and citrus instead of salt and sugar.

Meal Plans for Vegan Children

> ➢ **Infants (6–12 months)**

Breakfast: Iron-fortified cereal mixed with breast milk or formula, plus mashed banana.

Lunch: pureed lentils with sweet potato and spinach.

Dinner: Mashed avocado and soft-cooked quinoa.

Snacks include smooth nut butter diluted with water on soft bread and cooked carrot sticks.

> ➢ **Toddlers (ages 1-3 years)**

Breakfast: oatmeal with almond milk, blueberries, and chia seeds.

Lunch: Soft tofu cubes served with steaming broccoli and brown rice.

Dinner: lentil stew with carrots, peas, and whole-grain bread.

Snacks: Apple slices with hummus and whole grain crackers.

➤ **Preschoolers (ages 3-5 years)**

Breakfast smoothie made with spinach, banana, almond milk, and flaxseed.

Lunch: Chickpea salad with cucumber, tomato, and lemon-tahini dressing.

Dinner: Stir-fried tofu with mixed vegetables and quinoa.

Snacks include sliced bell peppers with guacamole, trail mix with nuts, and dried fruit.

Recipes for breakfast, lunch, dinner, and snacks

Breakfast: Banana Oat Pancakes

Ingredients: one ripe banana, one cup rolled oats, one cup almond milk, one teaspoon baking powder, and one teaspoon vanilla extract.

Instructions:

- Combine all ingredients and blend until smooth.

- Preheat a nonstick skillet over medium heat.

- Pour the batter into tiny pancakes.

- Cook until bubbles appear, then turn and finish until golden brown.

Lunch: Chickpea Avocado Salad

Ingredients: 1 can chickpeas (drained and rinsed), 1 diced avocado, 1 small cucumber, 1 chopped tomato, 2 tbsp lemon juice, salt, and pepper to taste.

Instructions:

- In a large mixing basin, add chickpeas, avocado, cucumber, and tomato.

- Drizzle with lemon juice, then season with salt and pepper.

- Toss gently until combined.

Dinner

Lentils and Vegetable Stew

Ingredients: 1 cup lentils, 2 diced carrots, 2 diced celery stalks, 1 chopped onion, 2 minced garlic cloves, 1 can diced tomatoes, 4 cups vegetable broth, 1 tsp thyme, and salt and pepper to taste.

Instructions:

- In a large pot, cook the onion and garlic until softened.

- Add the carrots and celery and simmer for 5 minutes.

- Stir in the lentils, tomatoes, broth, and thyme.

- Bring to a boil, then reduce heat and simmer for 30-40 minutes, or until the lentils are cooked.

- Season with salt and pepper.

Snacks

Energy Balls

Ingredients: 1 cup pitted dates, 1 cup oatmeal, 2 tablespoons chia seeds, 2 tablespoons almond butter, and 1 tablespoon chocolate powder.

Instructions:

- In a food processor, puree the dates until smooth.

- Combine oats, chia seeds, almond butter, and chocolate powder.

- Blend until thoroughly blended.

- Roll the mixture into small balls and chill for at least 30 minutes before serving.

Ensuring Adequate Nutrient Intake

> **Iron**

Iron is essential for oxygen transfer in the blood and maintaining overall energy levels. Plant sources of iron include:

- Legumes include lentils, chickpeas, and beans (black and kidney beans).

- Tofu and Tempeh: Soy products are high in iron.

- Dark leafy greens include spinach, kale, and Swiss chard.

- Nuts and seeds include pumpkin seeds, sesame seeds, and cashews.

- Whole grains include quinoa, brown rice, and fortified cereals.

- Dried fruits include apricots, raisins, and prunes.

Enhancing Iron Absorption:

Combine iron-rich foods with vitamin C-rich foods (citrus fruits, bell peppers, strawberries) to improve absorption.

Avoid taking iron inhibitors (such as tea, coffee, and dairy) in close proximity to iron-rich foods.

> **Zinc**

Zinc promotes immunological activity and cell repair. Plant-based zinc sources include:

- Legumes include chickpeas, lentils, and beans.

- Nuts and seeds include pumpkin seeds, sunflower seeds, and hemp seeds.

- Whole grains include oatmeal, quinoa, and brown rice.

- Nutritional yeast: Frequently supplemented with zinc.

- Vegetables include spinach, mushrooms, and broccoli.

> **Calcium**

Calcium is necessary for bone health, muscle function, and nerve transmission. Plant-based calcium sources include:

- Fortified plant milks include almond milk, soy milk, and oat milk.

- Tofu: particularly calcium-set tofu.

- Dark leafy greens include collards, kale, and bok choy.

- Broccoli and Brussels Sprouts are good vegetable sources.

- Tahini contains almonds and sesame seeds.

- Fortified foods include orange juice and cereals.

➢ **Vitamin D**

Vitamin D improves calcium absorption and bone health. Vitamin D can be obtained from plants using the following methods:

- Sunlight: Regular, moderate exposure to sunlight allows the body to create vitamin D.

- Fortified foods include plant milks, orange juice, and cereals.

- Mushrooms, particularly those exposed to UV radiation (e.g., Maitake, Portobello).

- Supplementation: Vitamin D2 is derived from plants, whilst D3 can be obtained from lichens, making it suitable for vegans.

➢ **Omega-3 Fatty Acids**

Omega-3 fatty acids are essential for brain development, particularly in newborns and toddlers. Plant-based sources include the following:

- Chia seeds are high in alpha-linolenic acid (ALA).

- Flaxseeds can be ground or in the form of oil.

- Hemp seeds are a good source of ALA.

- Walnuts contain a considerable quantity of ALA.

> **Algal oil**

Algal oil, a direct source of DHA (docosahexaenoic acid) and EPA (eicosapentaenoic acid), is commonly utilized in vegan supplements.

> **Vitamin B12:**

Vitamin B12 is required for nerve function, red blood cell formation, and DNA synthesis. Deficiency can cause anemia, tiredness, and neurological problems.

Plant-Based Sources and Supplements

Foods fortified with B12 include nutritional yeast, plant milks, morning cereals, and meat replacements.

Supplements: Because there are few reliable plant-based sources of B12, vegans should take a supplement.

Types: Cyanocobalamin and methylcobalamin

Dosage: The recommended daily amount varies by age, but people require approximately 2.4 micrograms per day. Consult a healthcare professional for specific guidance.

A well-balanced and nutritious plant-based diet can be maintained by eating these nutrient-rich foods and acknowledging the significance of supplementing when needed to support general health and development.

CHAPTER SIX

Plant-Based Myths and Facts

Myth:

Plant-based diets lack sufficient protein.

Fact:

A well-planned plant-based diet can provide all the essential amino acids and adequate protein levels. Foods like beans, lentils, tofu, tempeh, quinoa, and nuts are excellent protein sources.

Myth:

You need to combine proteins at each meal to get a complete protein.

Fact:

As long as a variety of plant foods are consumed over the course of a day, your body can obtain all the essential amino acids needed. The concept of protein combining at each meal is outdated.

Myth:

Animal protein is superior to plant protein.

Fact:

Plant proteins can be just as beneficial as animal proteins. They also come with added health benefits such as fiber, vitamins, minerals, and antioxidants, while being lower in saturated fat and cholesterol.

Facts

Plant-based protein can support muscle growth and repair.

Athletes and bodybuilders can meet their protein needs through plant-based sources. Pea protein, soy protein, and hemp protein powders are popular supplements.

Fact:

Variety is key to getting complete protein on a plant-based diet.

Consuming a diverse range of plant-based foods ensures that you receive all essential amino acids.

Fact:

Some plant-based proteins are complete proteins.

Foods like quinoa, buckwheat, chia seeds, and soy products contain all nine essential amino acids.

Identifying Food Allergies and Sensitivities

Symptoms: Look for symptoms such as hives, swelling, digestive issues, respiratory problems, and anaphylaxis after eating certain foods.

Testing: Consult a healthcare provider for skin tests, blood tests, or elimination diets to identify specific food allergies or sensitivities.

Managing Allergies

- Eliminate the allergen from the diet entirely. Read labels carefully to avoid cross-contamination.

- Use allergy-friendly substitutes. For example, use almond milk or oat milk instead of cow's milk, and chickpea flour or applesauce as egg substitutes.

- Have an action plan in case of accidental exposure, including the use of antihistamines or an epinephrine auto-injector (EpiPen).

Managing Sensitivities

- Moderation: Some people with sensitivities can tolerate small amounts of the problematic food. Monitor and adjust intake accordingly.

- Diet Adjustment: Gradually reintroduce the food in small amounts to determine tolerance levels, under the guidance of a healthcare provider.

Dealing with Picky Eaters

Strategies to Encourage Healthy Eating

- Provide a variety of foods in different colors, shapes, and textures to make meals more appealing.

- Let children help with meal planning, shopping, and cooking to increase their interest in trying new foods.

- Children are more likely to try new foods if they see their parents and siblings eating and enjoying them.

- Serve small portions to avoid overwhelming the child. They can always ask for more.

- Arrange food in fun shapes or patterns, use colorful plates, or create a themed meal to make eating more exciting.

- Repeatedly offer new foods without pressuring the child to eat them. It may take several exposures before a child accepts a new food.

- Establish regular meal and snack times to create a predictable routine.

- Turn off screens and create a calm, focused eating environment.

- Praise and encourage the child when they try new foods, rather than using negative reinforcement or punishments.

By understanding these aspects of nutrition and behavior, you can effectively support a healthy, balanced diet and create a positive eating environment for children and adults alike.

Promoting Physical Activity

Advantages of Engaging in Physical Activity

Physical Health: Enhances cardiovascular fitness, promotes robust skeletal structure and muscular development, and facilitates weight management.

Mental health: Alleviates symptoms of anxiety and depression, boosts mood, and optimizes cognitive performance.

Social Skills: Offers children the chance to acquire skills in teamwork, cooperation, and communication.

Methods to Promote Physical Activity

- Set a positive example for others to follow: Exemplify good behavior by actively engaging in physical activity yourself and including your family in the process.

- Ensure an engaging experience: Opt for activities that are pleasurable and diverse to sustain children's interest. Some examples of activities are playing tag, riding bikes, or dancing.

- Integrate Play: Employ play-oriented exercises such as hide and seek, obstacle courses, and sports to encourage physical activity.

- Restrict the amount of time dedicated to using televisions, computers, and mobile devices in order to promote engagement in more physically active hobbies.

- Create a consistent schedule that incorporates regular physical exercises, such as stretching in the morning, participating in sports after school, or going on hikes during the weekends.

Activities Suitable for Specific Age Groups

- ➤ For infants, it is beneficial to engage in activities such as tummy time, crawling games, and interactive play with toys.

- ➤ Toddlers can engage in locomotion activities such as walking, running, climbing, and engaging in ball play.

- ➤ Preschoolers can engage in activities such as riding tricycles or bikes, swimming, and playing on the playground.

- ➤ For school-aged children, suitable activities include organized sports, martial arts, dance lessons, and engaging in family activities such as hiking.

➢ Establish a tranquil bedtime routine by engaging in activities that promote relaxation, such as reading a book, indulging in a warm bath, or listening to soothing music.

➢ Prevent your kids from consuming stimulants such as caffeine and heavy meals prior to going to bed.

➢ Minimize the amount of time spent looking at screens by at least one hour prior to going to sleep.

➢ Optimize the sleep environment by ensuring that the bedroom is maintained at a low temperature, devoid of light, and free from any noise disturbances. Utilize a mattress and pillows that provide optimal comfort.

➢ Promote Daytime Physical Activity: Ensure that your kids engage in ample physical activity during the day to enhance their quality of sleep at night.

Importance of Optimal Sleep Habits

- ➢ Physical Health: Enhances the process of growth, fortifies the immune system, and facilitates the body's healing and restoration.

- ➢ Cognitive Function: Improves memory, acquisition of knowledge, focus, and ability to solve problems.

- ➢ Enhances emotional well-being by positively influencing mood and regulating emotions.

- ➢ For infants aged 4-12 months, it is recommended that they sleep for 12-16 hours within a 24-hour period, which includes both daytime naps and nighttime sleep.

- ➢ Toddlers between the ages of 1 and 2 require around 11 to 14 hours of sleep during a 24-hour period, which includes both daytime naps and nighttime sleep.

- ➢ Preschool-aged children, specifically those between the ages of 3 and 5, should sleep for a duration of 10 to 13 hours during a 24-hour period, which includes time spent napping.

- ➢ For children between the ages of 6 and 12, it is recommended that they get 9 to 12 hours of sleep per night.

- ➢ Adolescents aged 13 to 18 should aim to get 8 to 10 hours of sleep per night.

CHAPTER SEVEN

Significance of Emotional and Social Development

- Emotional intelligence aids in the comprehension and regulation of children's own emotions, as well as the recognition and empathy towards the emotions of others.

- Social skills are crucial for establishing and maintaining relationships, fostering cooperation, and facilitating effective communication.

- Self-esteem is enhanced by positive emotional and social growth, which leads to a strong sense of self-worth and confidence.

Methods to Facilitate Emotional and Social Growth

- Behavior Modeling: Exhibit constructive emotional expression and effective coping mechanisms.

- Promote open communication by encouraging your kids to express their emotions and actively listening to them without imposing any form of criticism or judgment.

- Assist your kids in acquiring techniques for effectively handling stress, such as practicing deep breathing, engaging in journaling, or seeking guidance from a reliable adult.

- Utilize positive reinforcement by commending your child for effectively expressing their emotions in a healthy manner and resolving problems in a constructive way.

- Ensure unwavering assistance: Establish a secure and nurturing setting that fosters children's confidence in sharing their feelings.

- Promote Social Interaction: Facilitate occasions for youngsters to engage with their peers through playdates, collective activities, and local community events.

- Engage your kids in role-playing exercises to facilitate the acquisition of social skills such as sharing, turn-taking, and dispute resolution.

- Promote empathy: Educate children on comprehending and valuing the viewpoints and emotions of others.

- Establish guidelines and limitations: Create explicit guidelines for appropriate conduct and ensure their consistent implementation.

- Facilitate opportunities for teamwork: Engage your child in collective endeavors and team-based sports to cultivate their abilities in collaboration and communication.

By integrating these activities into everyday routines, you may cultivate a comprehensive environment that encourages physical exercise, promotes healthy sleep patterns, and supports emotional and social growth for both children and adults.

Advantages of Adopting a Vegan Lifestyle

- Plant-based diets result in decreased emissions of carbon dioxide, methane, and nitrous oxide in comparison to diets that mostly consist of animal products, hence reducing greenhouse gas emissions.

- The conservation of water resources is promoted by the production of plant-based foods, which often necessitate less water compared to the breeding of animals for meat and dairy.

- Plant-based diets require less area for agricultural cultivation than cattle production.

- By diminishing the demand for animal products, we can safeguard habitats and endangered species by reducing deforestation and overgrazing.

- Plant agriculture generally leads to lower levels of pollution caused by manure and chemical runoff in comparison to extensive animal production.

Concrete Measures

- Minimize Food Waste: Strategize meal planning, repurpose leftovers, and compost food remnants.

- Purchase products from nearby sources and during their respective seasons: Aid local agricultural producers and diminish the environmental impact related to the transportation of food.

- Opt for Organic: Organic farming methods are frequently more sustainable and less detrimental to the environment.

- Opt for whole foods instead of overly processed alternatives to save energy and resource consumption.

Foundations of Conscious and Mindful Parenting

- Promote mindfulness in children by fostering their awareness of their thoughts, emotions, and behaviors.

- Encourage your child to cultivate mindfulness by directing their attention to the present moment, rather than allowing their thoughts to be consumed by concerns about the past or future.

- Encourage the adoption of a non-judgmental mindset towards oneself and others.

- Promote the development of empathy and benevolence towards oneself, others, and the environment.

- Implement age-appropriate mindfulness activities, such as practicing deep breathing, engaging in guided meditations, or participating in mindful walking.

- Promote daily introspection by engaging in journaling or discussing one's experiences and emotions from the day.

- Decrease interruptions by setting a limit on the amount of time spent using electronic devices and encouraging activities that need focused attention, such as reading or engaging in outdoor play.

- Engage in frequent conversations and actively demonstrate appreciation for the possessions and experiences they possess, cultivating a mindset of thankfulness.

- Educate your children on the significance of environmental stewardship by promoting recycling, practicing energy conservation, and minimizing trash.

- Allocate time in natural environments, foster your children's ability to carefully examine and value their surroundings.

- Utilize many forms of artistic expression, such as visual art, music, and imaginative play, to facilitate children's self-expression and promote their mindfulness.

- Engage in mindful eating by consciously tasting food, consuming it at a leisurely pace, and actively addressing the sensory aspects of meals.

- Introduce yoga or other forms of mindful movement exercises to facilitate children's connection with their bodies and thoughts.

By incorporating these principles and instructions into everyday life, you can contribute to the development of compassionate, empathic, ecologically aware, and attentive children.

END